Sameh ACHOURA
Kaouther SOMRANI

Lumbar disc herniation in adolescents

Sameh ACHOURA
Kaouther SOMRANI

Lumbar disc herniation in adolescents

Clinical features and treatment methods

ScienciaScripts

Imprint

Any brand names and product names mentioned in this book are subject to trademark, brand or patent protection and are trademarks or registered trademarks of their respective holders. The use of brand names, product names, common names, trade names, product descriptions etc. even without a particular marking in this work is in no way to be construed to mean that such names may be regarded as unrestricted in respect of trademark and brand protection legislation and could thus be used by anyone.

Cover image: www.ingimage.com

This book is a translation from the original published under ISBN 978-620-6-71123-0.

Publisher:
Sciencia Scripts
is a trademark of
Dodo Books Indian Ocean Ltd. and OmniScriptum S.R.L publishing group

120 High Road, East Finchley, London, N2 9ED, United Kingdom
Str. Armeneasca 28/1, office 1, Chisinau MD-2012, Republic of Moldova, Europe
Printed at: see last page
ISBN: 978-620-8-06139-5

TABLE OF CONTENTS

INTRODUCTION

A herniated disc is when part of the nucleus pulposus (the pulpy nucleus of the intervertebral disc) passes through the annulus fibrosus (the annulus fibrosus) into the spinal canal behind it. This nucleus can then compress the nerve root.

It is often the result of degenerative involution of the intervertebral disc. It leads to deformation or rupture of the posterior common vertebral ligament. This leads to a reduction in the calibre of the vertebral canal or the conjugation canal, responsible for the compression of one or more nerve roots, hence the appearance of the clinical symptom: lumbosciatica, which is the leading cause of consultation in neurosurgery, reflecting the disco-radicular conflict.

It occurs mainly in the last lumbar vertebrae, as a result of the high levels of pressure they have to withstand during forceful movements or trauma (1).

HDL is a rare cause of morbidity in adolescents. Its pathogenesis has not yet been fully elucidated.However, genetic, traumatic and biomechanical causes have been reported as factors in the development of HDL in under-19s.

HDL in adults is a frequent pathology. It is caused by degeneration and dehydration of the disc.

Our study focuses on HDL in patients under 19 years of age. Its incidence worldwide is 4 per 10,000.

In this case, the disc is well hydrated. HDL in adolescents is therefore considered to be a totally distinct pathology from that commonly observed in adults, due to its pathogenesis and natural history. specific. The age at which epidemiological changes occur is not yet well defined.

Due to the rarity of this condition in people under 19, it is often diagnosed late.

This prompted us to make it the subject of a study with the following objectives:

- To identify the clinical and paraclinical features of herniated lumbar discs in adolescents that distinguish them from those in adults.

- Determine its treatment and its prognosis.

METHODS

1. Equipment:

This is a retrospective cross-sectional descriptive study of 15 patients under 19 years of age operated on for HDL in the neurosurgery department of the Hôpital Militaire Principal d'Instruction de Tunis (from January 2012 to December 2019).

Inclusion criteria :

Our study included all patients with HDL who had undergone surgery in our department during the study period, and whose age was less than 19 years, regardless of sex.

Non-inclusion criteria :

This study did not include :

- Patients operated on for HDL and aged over 19.

- Patients under 19 years of age with non-operated HDL

- Files that cannot be used or are incomplete.

- Patients operated on outside this period.

A total of 15 cases meeting the inclusion and exclusion criteria were selected.

2. Methods :

All patients were treated and followed at the neurosurgery department of the Hôpital Militaire Principal d'Instruction in Tunis. Clinical data were collected using information contained in :

- The department's patient files.

- Consultation forms.

- Surgical reports.

The data collected made it possible to study, for each patient :

- Frequency and epidemiological characteristics: age, sex, personal and family history, physical activity.

- The clinical and paraclinical characteristics of HDL.

- Management of HDL: indication for surgery, surgical technique.

- Immediate and long-term post-operative outcomes: length of hospital stay, improvement in symptoms.

Declaration of interests

We declare that we have no conflicts of interest in relation to our study.

3. Statistical study :

The data was entered into an EXCEL file.

In order to compare our results with those in the literature, we carried out a bibliographic search using Pub Med, ScienceDirect and Google Scholar using the following key words: lumbar disc herniation, adolescent, diagnosis, surgery.

RESULTS

1. Epidemiology :

Age at the time of the operation :

The age of patients at the time of surgery ranged from 14 to 18 years.

The mean age was 16.6 years.

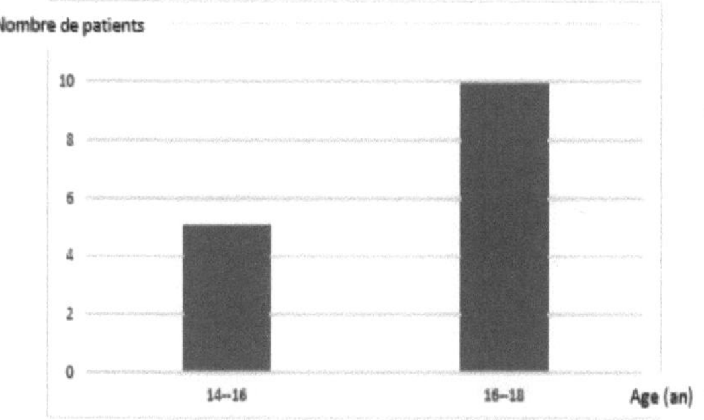

Figure 1: Age distribution of patients

Gender :

There was a predominance of males, with 10 males and 5 females.

The sex ratio obtained was 2. The following diagram shows this

distribution.

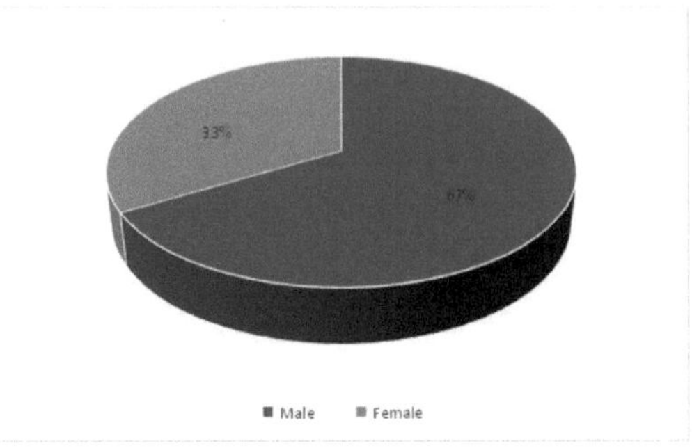

Figure 2: Breakdown of patients by sex

Particular family history :

Two of the patients had a family history of HDL in one of their parents, one of whom underwent a surgical cure.

Personal history :

Only one patient had iron deficiency anaemia

Habits and sporting activity :

Three of the patients took part in regular sporting activities. Two did bodybuilding and one did gymnastics.

2. Clinical study :

Time to positive diagnosis :

The time between the onset of symptoms and positive diagnosis varied between 1 and 6 months, with an average of 4.2 months.

Notion of lumbar trauma :

This notion was found in 6 patients, including 2 cases of sporting accidents, 2 cases of domestic accidents and 2 cases of road accidents.

Reason for consultation :

In all cases, patients consulted for unilateral, monoradicular mechanical lumbosciatica of type L5 in 12 cases and type S1 in 3 cases, right in 9 cases and left in 6 cases. 4 patients suffered from intermittent radicular claudication with a reduction in walking perimeter. None of the patients had vesicosphincter disorders.

Neurological examination :

Spinal syndrome was noted in all patients.

-A pseudo-scoliotic analgesic attitude in 9 patients.

Spinal stiffness in all these patients, defined by a hand-to-ground distance > 10 cm. This distance was > 20 cm in 6 cases.

Lasègue's sign was found unilaterally in all patients. It was <30° in 6 patients.

Hypoesthesia of the L5 and S1 territories was found in 3 patients.

Abolition of achilles ROTs was found in 2 patients.

No motor deficits or anaesthesia in the saddle were found.

General review :

A lanky morphotype was found in 6 patients, 4 of whom were boys.

The BMI varied between 18 and 27.5.

Duration of medical treatment :

The duration of the medical treatment, which included analgesics, anti-inflammatories and muscle relaxants, as well as a healthy lifestyle and motor rehabilitation, varied between 2 months and 2 years, with an average of 10 months.

Additional tests:

Lumbar CT :

Lumbar CT scans were performed in all patients, and lumbar MRI was performed in 6 cases.

They showed:

• 3 cases of double HDL: L4-L5 and L5-S1 (Figure 3)

• 4 cases of narrow lumbar canal aggravated by HDL L4 -L5

• 5 cases of simple L4-L5 HDL

• 3 cases of simple L5-S1 HDL

• Avulsion of the posterior marginal listel in 4 cases 6 of these hernias were particularly large.

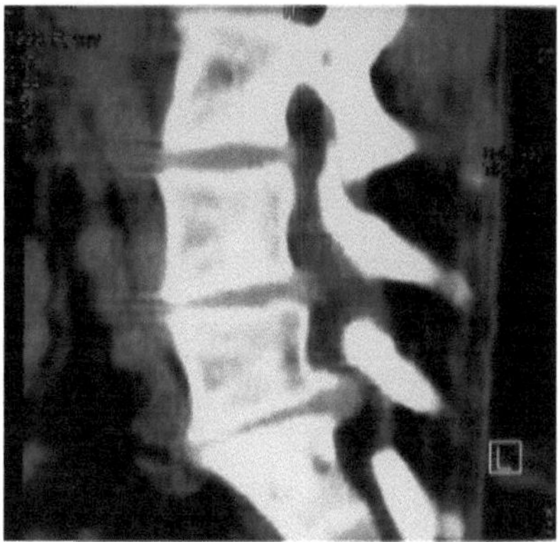

Figure 3.b

Figure 3.a

Figure 3: Lumbar CT scan

a- Sagittal section showing double HDL L4-L5 and L5-S1

b- Axial section showing double HDL L4-L5 and L5-S1 medial and paramedial left

Lumbar MRI :

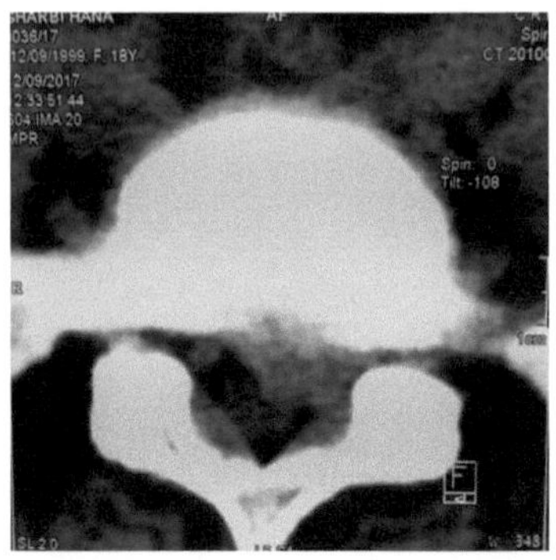

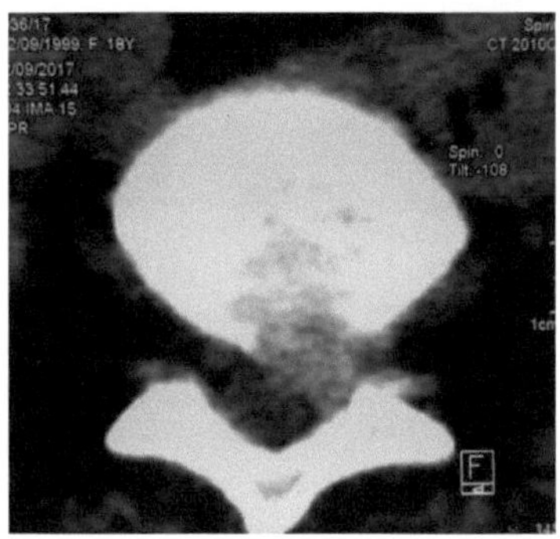

It was carried out in 6 cases (Figure 4).

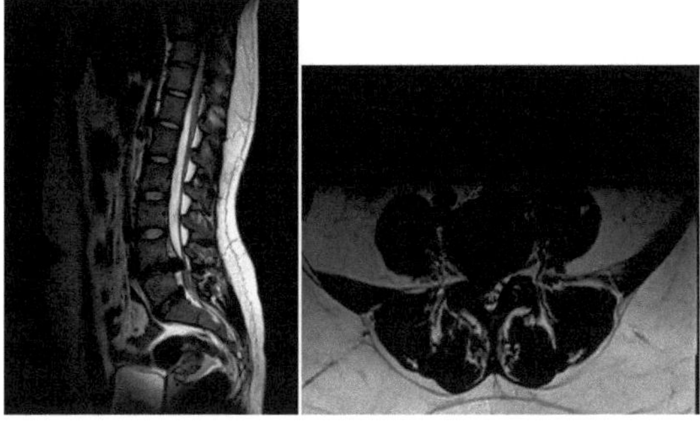

Figure 4.a

Figure 4.b

Figure 4: Lumbar MRI:

a- T2 sagittal section showing a large L4-L5 HDL

b- Axial T2 section showing a voluminous L4-L5 median and right paramedian HDL

3. Surgical treatment :

In our series, all patients underwent surgery because their sciatica was resistant to medical treatment.

Surgical technique :

• A single-stage unilateral interlaminal approach was proposed in 9 cases and a 2-stage approach in 2 cases.

• The operation consisted of removal of the hernia combined with careful discectomy.

• 4 cases of narrow lumbar canal aggravated by HDL benefited from an interspinous approach.

Intraoperative findings :

In all patients, the herniated disc was found to be particularly soft and the disc was well hydrated.

In 6 patients, the herniated disc was particularly large.

4. Post-operative course: Length of hospital stay :

The average length of stay was 48 hours.

Evolution of symptoms :

Patient follow-up ranged from 6 months to 24 months.

There was a marked improvement in sciatica in all cases. Four of the patients still had mechanical low back pain.

No impact on spinal statics was noted during the follow-up period.

No cases of recurrence were reported.

Surgical complications :

Only one case of dural breach (sutured intraoperatively) was reported in our series. It was not complicated by CSF leakage or meningitis.

No other complications of an infectious nature or haematoma at the site were reported.

Rehabilitation and healthy living:

All patients underwent motor rehabilitation starting 1 month after surgery and continuing for 3 months, with 3 sessions per week. It included strengthening the erector spinae muscles and gait re-education.

DISCUSSION

Although lumbar disc herniation is a frequent pathology in adults, it is rare in subjects under the age of 19. Our study set out to determine the aetiopathogenic, clinical and paraclinical characteristics of HDL in adolescents, and to emphasise the importance of early and specific management. However, our study is limited by the relatively small number of cases and its retrospective nature.

1. Theoretical background :

Anatomy :

The intervertebral disc :

As the main link between the lumbar vertebrae, the IVD not only resists gravity and complex mechanical stresses, but also ensures multidirectional mobility of the lumbar spine. This fibrocartilage has a highly variable shape corresponding to that of the vertebral plates. In the lumbar region, the thickness of the IVD varies from 10 to 15 mm and increases from L1-L2 to L4-L5. The high disc index (ratio between the height of the IVD and the vertebral body equal to 1/5) favours mobility. The IVD is thicker anteriorly than posteriorly, helping to form the physiological lumbar lordosis. It adheres to the vertebral plates and the common anterior and posterior vertebral ligaments.

It is an avascular structure with little innervation in the normal state, and consists of two parts (Figure 5):

 The nucleus pulposus or nucleus pulposus: located in the centre of the disc and whose boundaries with the annulus fibrosus are not very clear. It is a gel rich in water (80%) and proteoglycans.

 The annulus fibrosus or annulus: this corresponds to the peripheral part of the IVD, made up of concentric lamellae whose fibres are very close together and oblique, which allows them to slide in relation to each other, enabling the disc to resist tensile, compressive or torsional stress.

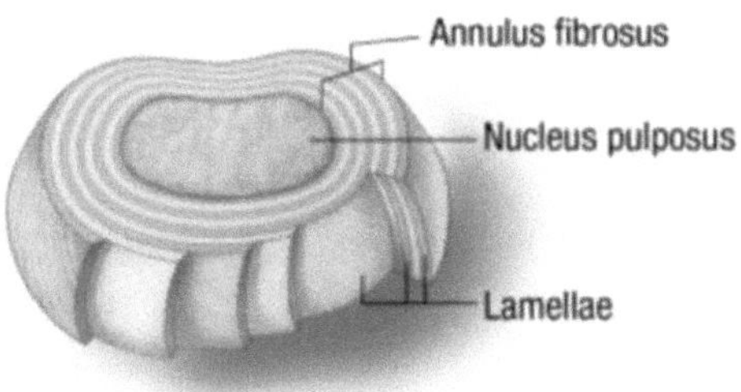

Figure 5: The intervertebral disc (2)

Lumbar spinal nerves :

Contained in the dural sac with the other meningeal envelopes and the CSF, the lumbar spinal nerves provide sensory-motor innervation of the two lower limbs (Figure 6). The greater sciatic nerve contains fibres from the 4th and 5th lumbar nerves and the 1st to 3rd sacral nerves. It is flattened in shape and 10 to 15 mm wide at its origin. It runs downwards, first in the gluteal region and then in the posterior region of the thigh. It divides at the popliteal fossa into two terminal branches, the common fibular nerve (or external popliteal sciatic nerve) and the tibial nerve (or internal popliteal sciatic nerve). The L5 and S1 roots form the bulk of the fibres making up the sciatic nerve:

♣ The L5 roots: arise opposite the middle part of the spinous process of D12.

♣ S1 roots: originate below the spinous process of L2. They descend inside the dural sac, then leave it by perforating the dura mater and enter the epidural space to reach the foramen magnum, from where they exit the spine.

♣ Along its path, the root describes two sections:

o An intradural portion, which travels among the roots of the cauda equina until it emerges from the dura mater, behind the posterior surface of the L4-L5 disc for the L5 roots and at the level of the inferior edge of the L5-S1 disc for the S1 roots.

o An extradural portion, divided into 3 segments:

* The retro-discal segment: forms the interdiscoligamentary pathway. This is where the roots are subject to compression.

* The pedicle segment: at this level, the root is located between the vertebral body at the front, the pedicle at the outside and the superior articular joint at the back.

* The foraminal segment: this is where the spinal ganglion is found. Only the upper part of the foramen is in contact with the root. The lower part contains only fat and venous anastomoses (3).

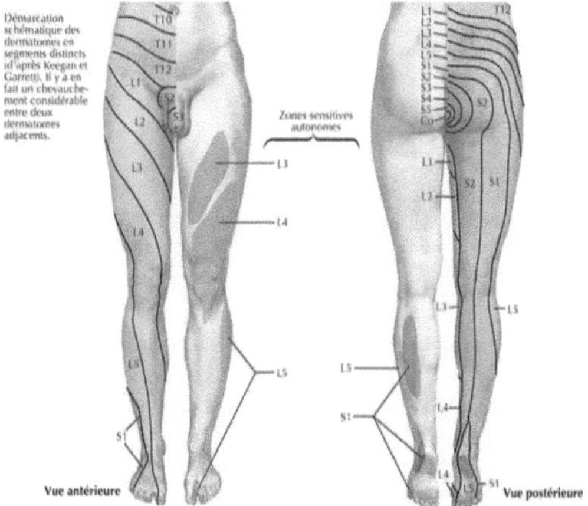

Figure 6: Dermatomas of the lower limb (4)

Pathophysiology :

Disc damage :

In adults, disc deterioration is mainly due to ageing, which is accompanied by changes in structure, composition and vascularisation. These changes are responsible for the weakening of the disc. Later on, radial fissures will form, the appearance of which seems to coincide with the clinical manifestations. In adolescents, HDL is often post-traumatic; violent lumbar spinal trauma is responsible for intra-disc hyperpressure by a flexion-compression mechanism which is responsible for rupture of the posterior part of the annulus fibrosus (5). The rarity of HDL in in adolescents is explained by the nature of the IVD, which is more hydrated than that of adults (6).

Hernia :

There is no modification of the nucleus without advanced abnormalities of the annulus. In lumbar spinal trauma, rupture of the posterior part of the annulus disc is associated with herniation of part of the nucleus backwards, compressing either the dural sheath and the cord, or the lateral nerve roots. On its path, the nucleus will encounter two superimposed barriers:

- The first consists of the vertical fibres of the annulus fibrosus of the disc.

- The second, more resistant, is formed by the fibres of the posterior common vertebral ligament, which is more resistant in the medial part.

In the first stage, of varying duration, the repressed nucleus will distend the annulus fibrosus and push back the posterior common vertebral ligament: this is the stage of disc distension, which is expressed clinically by pure low back pain, lumbosacralgia or attacks of lumbago. In a second stage, distension by the nucleus of what remains of the fibrous ring and the posterior common vertebral ligament will produce a posterior bulge, often transferred to the lateral parts of this ligament: this is the stage of disc protrusion. The disco-radicular conflict is then triggered. At this stage, as at the following stage, the pressure of the nucleus tends to be reduced by the homolateral and posterior disc bâillement. The same applies when the nucleus is reintegrated. The root itself is the site of an "inflammatory radiculitis" resulting from the compression. In a third stage, the fibrous ring will break, the fibrocartilaginous sequestration and part of the nucleus will be enucleated and herniate, lodging in front of the posterior common vertebral ligament: this is disc sequestration. The herniation becomes irreducible. At this stage, as with at the next stage, discoradicular impingement may be very acute. Similarly, radicular ischaemia due to compression may occur, leading to a motor deficit. This is the paralysing form. In the fourth stage, the posterior common vertebral ligament may itself be perforated and the sequestrum becomes externalized: this is the stage of disc exclusion, the symptoms and course of which vary according to the volume of the sequestrum (3).

Pain mechanisms :

Since the demonstration of the link between herniated discs and sciatica, it has been accepted that radicular compression by a herniated disc is the cause of sciatica, but it is now accepted that there are chemical factors in addition to the mechanical component. The clinical arguments in favour of the "chemical" theory are :

- failure rates for disc surgery

- the existence of large asymptomatic disc herniations

- the existence of severe radiculalgia without radicular compression

- the poor correlation between the severity of neurological symptoms and the size of the herniated disc

- the often favourable outcome after conservative treatment

- Experimental arguments also support this theory:

- The capacity for spontaneous resorption of the herniated disc

- Immunogenicity of the intervertebral disc

- the presence of inflammatory mediators within the disc. The current physiopathological theory incriminates pro-inflammatory substances secreted by the nucleus pulposus (NP) which, in order to cause radiculalgia, must be associated with prior or simultaneous mechanical root attack (3). Animal experiments have shown that NP can, without mechanical compression, induced functional and structural abnormalities in the nerve root, and that these effects, which were more or less inhibited by methylprednisolone, diclofenac, indomethacin, doxycycline and cyclosporine, were generated by substances located on the surface of NP cells (3).

2. Epidemiological study: Frequency and incidence :

The incidence of lumbar disc herniation in subjects under 19 years of age is estimated at 5.5 cases per 100,000 people per year. In adults, it is 123.3 cases per 100,000 people (7). HDL in subjects under 19 represents 0.5 to 6.8% of all HDL (8).

Breakdown by age :

An American study of 87 children and adolescents operated on for HDL concluded that 51% were aged between 17 and 18, 46% were aged between 13 and 16 and 2.5% were aged under 12 (7). In our series, 33.3% of patients were aged between 14 and 16 years and 66.7% were aged between 16 and 18 years.

Gender :

There was a clear male predominance in all the series reported in the literature (9). The sex ratio varied. In a recent meta-analysis it was 1.5 (10). In our series it was 2.

Weight and size :

The relationship between obesity and HDL in adolescents is not yet well established. It is, however, associated with disc degeneration (10). In our series, only 13.3% of patients were overweight. Furthermore, in Kamoun's series (11), half the patients were thin and long-limbed, while only 18% were overweight. In our series, the percentage of long-limbed patients was 40%.

Sports activities :

Intense athletic activity 5 days a week or 20 hours a week is a factor in spondylolisthesis. Tennis players and weightlifters have been shown to develop disc pathologies and spondylolisthesis more frequently than the general population.

It is difficult to establish whether it is the spinal trauma or the sporting activity itself that is responsible for the HDL (10).

Lumbar trauma :

Trauma to the lumbar spine has been considered to be a factor favouring the onset of HDL in adolescents (10). This notion has been reported in several series at different percentages [33-100%] (12-15).

The rate of lumbar spinal trauma was 40% in our series.

Genetic factors :

13 to 57% of adolescents with HDL have a parent with the same condition (16). In our series this rate was 13%.

3. Clinical study :

Reason for consultation :

Clinical symptoms often differ from those seen in adults. Low back pain is often less intense than in adults (16). The combination of low back pain and sciatica is present in 58% of cases. for deORio et al (17) and in 70% of cases according to Ferrante et al (18). This lower frequency of functional symptoms in adolescents is linked to better tolerance of the nerve root. In our series, all patients presented with unilateral low back pain, associated in 26% of cases with intermittent radicular claudication.

Time to positive diagnosis :

It varied, with an average of 4.2 months. The delay in diagnosis sometimes observed was due to a lack of awareness of this pathology among adolescents. During this period, there was an impact on the teenagers' daily lives and schooling.

Neurological examination :

Spinal syndrome is usually more severe in adolescents than in adults. It is a more or less painful stiffness of the spine, which can erase the physiological lordosis, preventing normal anteflexion of the trunk. It is often accompanied by paravertebral contracture and lateral imbalance, or even a scoliotic attitude (16). Recent studies have concluded that HDL is most often lateralized on the convex side (87% of cases).(Scoliosis can lead to lameness (19) and may be a reason for consultation (16). For Liquois et al (20), spinal syndrome is a constant sign. In our series, the spinal syndrome was present in all patients. It was major in 60% of cases. For radicular syndrome, it appears that the Lasègue sign is more sensitive in adolescents than in adults (10). The Lasègue sign is found to be positive in 85% of cases according to Ginsburg et al (19) and in 92% of cases according to Ferrante et al (18). The Lasègue sign is most often severe (21). In our study, all patients had a Lasègue sign. It was tight in 40% of cases. Furthermore, according to the various series in the literature, the rate of motor deficit and ROT abnormalities is very low (10). In our series, hypoesthesia of the L5 and S1 territories was found in 20% of cases, abolition of achilles ROTs was found in 13% of cases and no patient presented a motor deficit.

Additional tests:

Lumbar CT :

This is the first-line examination.

The floors most frequently affected in adolescents are L4-L5 and L5-S1 (93% of cases) (10). The L4-L5 level is more frequent in adolescents than in adults (52% versus 41%) (10).

Lumbar CT scans were performed in all patients in our study. Double L4-L5 and L5-S1 HDL was found in 20% of cases, L4-L5 HDL in 60% of cases, associated with a narrow lumbar canal in 26% of cases, and single L5-S1 HDL in 20% of cases.

Avulsion of the posterior marginal listel was found in 26% of cases. In 40% of cases, the HDL was particularly large.

Avulsion of the posterior marginal listel corresponds to an acute or sub-acute detachment of the listel, of traumatic origin (20). This detachment may be visible from the age of 6, since ossification of the listel begins at this age and it fuses with the vertebral body from the age of 17. It is completely fused between the ages of 18 and 25 (20).

Lumbar MRI :

Although CT is the reference examination in the initial assessment of common sciatica, its inadequacy in terms of exploiting the intradural compartment means that MRI must be performed.

This allows :

♣ Analysis of hernial migration and associated ductal stenosis.

♣ Exploration of all the lumbar discs.

♣ Exploration of the intradural compartment.

In our series, lumbar MRI was performed in 40% of cases, in addition to the CT scan.

Treatment :

Medical treatment :

The first treatment to be implemented must be conservative. It involves a variable combination of rest, analgesics and anti-inflammatories, muscle relaxants, physiotherapy and a corset. The signs may regress, especially when the lesion is an isolated disc herniation without avulsion of the posterior marginal listel (18). For adults, the recommended duration of medical treatment is between 6 and 12 weeks (22). For adolescents, according to Fakouri (12), the average duration is 10.5 weeks. In these young patients, who are in the midst of their school, social and sporting activities, disabling and persistent low back pain can affect their performance.In addition, the duration of conservative treatment should be as short as possible, given the good results of surgical treatment and the greater impact on social life (12).All studies agree that HDL in adolescents responds less well to medical treatment than in adults (23). The duration of medical treatment was longer in our series, ranging from 2 months to 2 years, with an average of 10 months.

Surgical treatment :

It must treat the cause of the nerve compression and any associated abnormalities Narrow lumbar canal, instability.In the case of an isolated herniated disc, treatment should be limited to excision of the herniated fragment. In adolescents, the disc is very well hydrated. Complete disc curettage is difficult and exposes the patient to the risk of recurrence (18). In our study, we performed a complete excision of the herniated fragment and a cautious discectomy. In the case of avulsion of the posterior marginal listel, simple removal of the protruding fragment with preservation of the intervertebral disc is recommended by Liquois et al (20). Laminectomy should be avoided at all costs because of the risk of destabilising the adolescent (19). In our series, a single-stage interlaminal approach was proposed in 9 cases and a 2-stage approach in 2 cases. 4 cases of narrow lumbar canal aggravated by HDL benefited from an interspinous approach. Other surgical techniques have been reported in the literature. A study comparing discectomy with arthrodesis and discectomy alone showed no significant difference in functional results (23). Another Norwegian study compared conventional discectomy with microdiscectomy and concluded that there was no superiority for the latter technique (10).

Evolution :

Functional results :

After 1 to 2 years post-operatively, 4.5 to 14% of adolescents are dissatisfied (24), (25). Compared to adults, studies are not unanimous. In fact, a Swedish study and another Chinese study have shown that the percentage of adolescents with an improvement in low back pain was greater than in adults (15). In contrast, a Norwegian study showed no significant difference (10). In our study, patient follow-up varied between 6 and 24 months. There was a marked improvement in sciatica in all cases. Four of the patients retained mechanical low back pain.

Surgical complications :

There is general agreement in the literature that surgical complications are rare, occurring in less than 1% of cases. These complications are infectious or, more rarely, lead to haematoma at the site (10).

In our series, only one case of dural breach was reported. It was not complicated by CSF leakage or meningitis. No other complications of an infectious nature or haematoma at the site were reported.

Risk of recurrence :

The risk of recurrence at the same level as the first operation is low: 3% for Zucker et al (26). On the other hand, the risk of recurrence is greater at adjacent levels: 8% for Ferrante et al (18). We did not observe any cases of recurrence in our series.

CONCLUSIONS

Lumbar disc herniation is a common pathology in adults but rare in adolescents, so diagnosis and treatment are sometimes delayed in people under 19.

Its aetiopathogenesis, clinical presentation and management are very specific to adolescents. This is why we decided to carry out this study.

This was a retrospective descriptive study of 15 patients operated on for HDL under 19 years of age in the neurosurgery department of the Hôpital Militaire Principal d'Instruction de Tunis over an 8-year period from January 2012 to December 2019.

The aim of our work was to determine the clinical and paraclinical features of lumbar disc herniation in adolescents that distinguish it from that in adults, and to determine the treatment methods and prognosis. In the course of our work, we were confronted with certain methodological difficulties, essentially due to the retrospective nature of our study, namely the lack of precision of some of the information in the medical records and operative reports. Our series included 10 boys and 5 girls. This male preponderance is consistent with the literature. The mean age at diagnosis was 16.6 years, with a predominance of 16-18 year olds.In terms of aetiopathogenic factors, a history of HDL in the parents was found in 13% of cases in our series. In the literature, it varied between 13 and 57%. The elongated morphotype was present in 40% of cases, in line with the data in the literature, where this percentage reached 50%. Lumbar spine trauma was found in 40% of our patients. According to the literature, this is considered to be a factor favouring the onset of HDL in adolescents. This notion has been reported in several series with different percentages [33-100%].

The reason for consultation was unilateral, monoradicular mechanical low back pain of the L5 type in 80% of cases and of the S1 type in 20%. 26% of patients suffered from intermittent radicular claudication. None of the patients had vesicosphincter disorders.

The spinal syndrome was major in 60% of cases and Lasègue's sign was severe in 40%. No motor deficit was found. Lumbar imaging revealed double L4-L5 and L5-S1 HDL in 20% of cases, L4-L5 HDL in 60% of cases, associated with a narrow lumbar canal in 26% of cases, and single L5-S1 HDL in 20% of cases.Avulsion of the posterior marginal listel was found in 26% of cases. In 40% of cases, the HDL was particularly large. This is in line with the literature, which has shown that the stages most frequently affected in adolescents are L4-L5 and L5-S1 (93% of cases) and that the L4-L5 stage is more frequent in adolescents than in adults.

The duration of medical treatment varied between 2 months and 2 years, with an average of 10 months. However, according to the latest recommendations in the literature, the duration of conservative treatment should be as short as possible (on average 10.5 weeks), given the good results of surgical treatment and the greater impact on social life.

In our series, a single-stage interlaminal approach was proposed in 60% of cases and a 2-stage approach in 13.3% of cases. 4 cases of narrow lumbar canal aggravated by HDL benefited from an interspinous approach.

We performed a complete excision of the herniated fragment combined with a careful discectomy. The disc material was well hydrated and abundant.

The surgical procedure must be the least damaging possible, respecting the means of spinal stability in a growing spine. Other surgical techniques have been reported in the literature. Discectomy with arthrodesis or microdiscectomy have not been shown to be superior to conventional discectomy. Post-operative follow-up ranged from 6 to 24 months. All patients showed an improvement in sciatica. This is in line with the very good results reported in the literature.

Our study was unable to determine precisely how quickly adolescents were able to return to school and to sport.

Patients were followed up for a maximum of 2 years. The long-term impact of HDL surgery during adolescence on spinal statics could not be studied. These shortcomings are due to the retrospective nature of the study. Unrecognised symptomatic HDL in adolescents can have significant functional and social repercussions. Early, specialised treatment is needed to ensure that the patient is operated on in good time. Physiotherapy plays a crucial role in improving post-operative functional results, preventing recurrence and enabling the patient to return to social and school life without delay.

REFERENCES

1. GOUPILLE, P1, [1] Rheumatology Department, CHU Trousseau, Tours, France. Causes of failed back surgery syndrome. Revue du rhumatisme (Ed française) 1996, Vol 63, Num 4, pp 255-260 ; ref : 40 ref ISSN 1169-8330 Domaine scientifique Orthopedics traumatology; Rheumatology.

2. Hooten WM, Cohen SP. Evaluation and Treatment of Low Back Pain. Mayo Clin Proc. Dec 2015;90(12):1699-718.

3. Mulleman D, Mammou S, Griffoul I, Watier H, Goupille P. Physiopathology of lumbosciatica caused by disc herniation. Rev Rhum. May 2006;73(5):453-61.

4. Themes UFO. 61: Skin anatomy | Medicine Key [Internet]. [cited 1 Oct 2020]. Available from: https://clemedicine.com/61-anatomie-cutanee/

5. 0100302TrduRachis.pdf [Internet]. [cited 1 Oct 2020]. Available from:

http://campus.neurochirurgie.fr/IMG/pdf/0100302TrduRachis.pdf

6. Kim D-K, Oh CH, Lee MS, Yoon SH, Park H, Park CO. Prevalence of Lumbar Disc Herniation in Adolescent Males in Seoul, Korea:

Prevalence of Adolescent LDH in Seoul, Korea. Korean J Spine. 2011;8(4):261.

7. Cahill KS, Dunn I, Gunnarsson T, Proctor MR. Lumbar microdiscectomy in pediatric patients: a large single-institution series. J Neurosurg Spine. Feb 2010;12(2):165-70.

8. Ozgen S, Konya D, Toktas OZ, Dagcinar A, Ozek MM. Lumbar Disc Herniation in Adolescence. Pediatr Neurosurg. 2007;43(2):77-81.

9. Silvers HR, Lewis PJ, Clabeaux DE, Asch HL. Lumbar Disc Excisions in Patients Under the Age of 21 Years: Spine. Nov 1994;19(21):2387-91.

10.Raghu ALB, Wiggins A, Kandasamy J. Surgical management of lumbar disc herniation in children and adolescents. Clin Neurol Neurosurg. Oct 2019;185:105486.

11.KAMOUN, N1; DZIRI, C1; BEN SALAH, F. Z1; DAGHFOUS, M. S2; HADIDANE, R1; LADEB, F3; DOUIK, M2; SLIMAN, N2. Lumbar disc herniation before 21 years old. Rachis (Clichy) 1997, Vol 9, Num 3, pp 131-136; ref: 22 ref. 1997;

12.Fakouri B, Nnadi C, Boszczyk B, Kunsky A, Cacciola F. When is the appropriate time for surgical intervention of the herniated lumbar disc in the adolescent? J Clin Neurosci. Sept 2009;16(9):1153-6.

13.Wang X, Zeng J, Nie H, Chen G, Li Z, Jiang H, et al. Percutaneous endoscopic interlaminar discectomy for pediatric lumbar disc herniation.Childs Nerv Syst. May 2014;30(5):897-902.

14.Montejo JD, Camara-Quintana JQ, Duran D, Rockefeller JM, Conine SB, Blaise AM, et al. Tubular approach to minimally invasive microdiscectomy for pediatric lumbar disc herniation. J Neurosurg Pediatr. May 2018;21(5):449-55.

15.Chen Y, Song R, Huang W, Chang Z. Percutaneous endoscopic discectomy in adolescent lumbar disc herniation: a 3- to 5-year study. J NeurosurgPediatr. Feb 2019;23(2):251-8.

16.CHATAIGNER, H1; ONIMUS, M1; GANGLOFF, S. LA HERNIE DISCALE DE L'ENFANT ET DE L'ADOLESCENT ASPECTS CLINIQUES ET THÉRAPEUTIQUES HERNIATED DISC IN CHILDHOOD CLINICAL AND THERAPEUTIC ASPECTS. Spine (Clichy) 1997, Vol 9, Num 4, pp 165-172, 7 p ; ref: 28 ref. 1997;

17.DeOrio JK, Bianco AJ. Lumbar disc excision in children and adolescents. J Bone Joint Surg Am. Sept 1982;64(7):991-6.

18.Ferrante L, Mastronardi L, Lunardi P, Puzzilli F, Fortuna A. Lumbar disc herniation in teenagers. Eur Spine J. June 1992;1(1):25-8.

19.Ginsburg GM, Bassett GS. Back Pain in Children and Adolescents: Evaluation and Differential Diagnosis: J Am Acad Orthop Surg. March 1997;5(2):67-78.

20.LIQUOIS, F1 ; DEMAY, P1 ; FILIPE, G1, [1] Department of Surgery Orthopédique et Réparatrice de l'Enfant, Hôpital Armand Trousseau, 26, avenue du Docteur Arnold Netter, 75571 Paris, France. Sciatica due to avulsion of the cartilaginous vertebral rim in children. Revue de chirurgie orthopédique et réparatrice de l'appareil moteur. 1997, Vol 83, Num 3, pp 210- 216; ref: 18 ref. 1997;

21.Takata K, Takahashi K. Hamstring tightness and sciatica in young patients with disc herniation. J Bone Joint Surg Br. March 1994;76(2):220-4.

22.Jacobs WCH, van Tulder M, Arts M, Rubinstein SM, van Middelkoop M, Ostelo R, et al. Surgery versus conservative management of sciatica due to a lumbar herniated disc: a systematic review. Eur Spine J. Apr 2011;20(4):513- 22.

23.Dang L, Liu Z. A review of current treatment for lumbar disc herniation in children and adolescents. Eur Spine J. 1 Feb 2010;19(2):205-14.

24.Strömqvist F, Strömqvist B, Jönsson B, Gerdhem P, Karlsson MK. Predictive outcome factors in the young patient treated with lumbar disc herniation surgery. J Neurosurg Spine. Oct 2016;25(4):448-55.

25.Lagerbäck T, Elkan P, Möller H, Grauers A, Diarbakerli E, Gerdhem P. An observational study on the outcome after surgery for lumbar disc herniation in adolescents compared with adults based on the Swedish Spine Register. Spine J. June 2015;15(6):1241-7.

26.Zucker L, Amacher AL, Eltomey A. Juvenile lumbar discs. Childs Nerv Syst. June 1987;3(2):125-7.

LUMBAR DISC HERNIATION IN ADOLESCENTS (ABOUT 15 CASES OPERATED)

ABSTRACT

Introduction :

Lumbar disc herniation is a frequent pathology in adults. It is associated with disc degeneration and dehydration. However, it is a rare condition in adolescents. Its ethiopathogeny, clinical presentation and managementare very specific in adolescents. The aim of our work was to determine the clinical, paraclinical characteristics of lumbar disc herniation in adolescents, its treatment and prognosis. Methods : We realized a retrospective descriptive study about 15 patients operated for LDH aged under 19 years at the neurosurgery department of the Military Hospital of Tunis during 8 years from January 2012 to December 2019.

Results :

The mean age at diagnosis was 16.6 year. There was a male predominance with a sex ratio of 2, and trauma was found in 40% of the cases. In all cases, patients consulted for unilateral and monoradicular mechanical lumbosciatica ,type L5 in 80% of cases and type S1 in 20% of cases associated with radicular claudication in 26% of cases. The rachidian syndrome was major in 60% of cases and the Lasegue sign was tight in 40% of cases. No motor deficit was found. Lumbar imaging found in 20% of cases a double LDH L4-L5 and L5-S1, in 60% of cases an LDH L4-L5 associated in 26% of cases with a narrow lumbar canal and in 20% of cases a single LDH L5-S1. Avulsion of the posterior marginal listel was found in 26% of cases. In 40% of the cases the LDH was particularly voluminous. The average duration of medical treatment was 10 months. In our series, a single-stage interlaminar approach was proposed in 60% of cases and a two-stage approach in 13.3% of cases.Four cases of narrow lumbar canal aggravated by LDH were treated with an interepinous approach. We performed a complete excision of the hernial fragment followed by a careful discectomy. The disc material was well hydrated and abundant. The duration of follow-up varied between 6 and 24 months. All patients showed an improvement in sciatica.

Conclusion:

Unknown symptomatic LDH in adolescent may have an important functional and social impact. An early and specialized management is necessary in order to make the surgical indication in time.

Key-words: lumbar disc herniation - adolescent - diagnosis - surgery

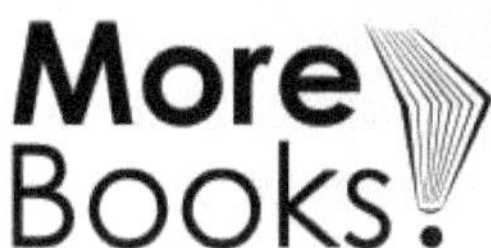
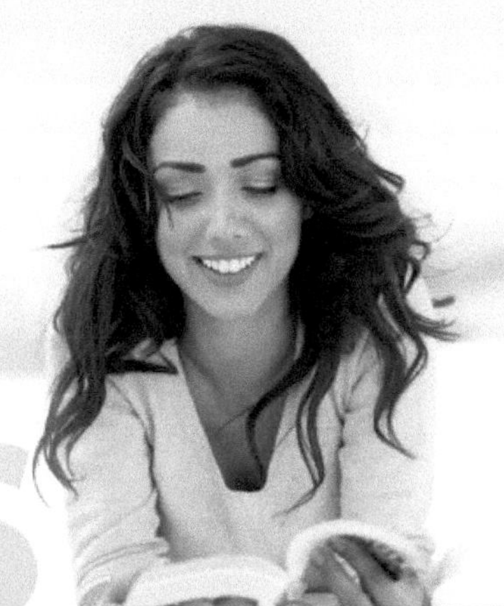

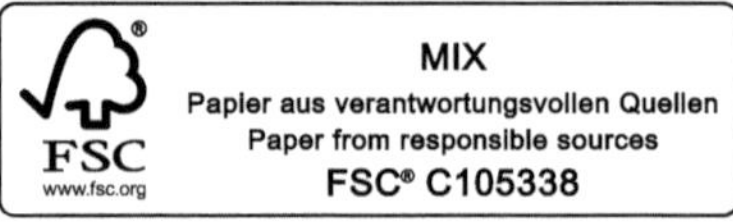

Printed by Books on Demand GmbH, Norderstedt / Germany